Clean Eating

Nourishing Superfood Salads For Effortless Weight
Management And Cleansing: Economical Superfood
Recipes For A Healthful Lifestyle

*(Enhance Your Weight Loss And Boost Your Energy Levels
Through Exquisite Clean Eating Recipes)*

Columbus Lambert

TABLE OF CONTENT

What Is Clean Eating?

Have you ever contemplated the journey of how the sustenance you consume is delivered to your table? What recommendations do you have for promoting your personal well-being, preserving natural resources, and ensuring environmental sustainability? How is it developed? Has it undergone genetic modification and is it treated with potentially harmful pesticides? Are animals reared in optimal conditions and provided with ethical treatment? What is the extent of fuel consumption required to transport your items to you? Does it emanate from your group or originate from a widespread global context?

Clean Eating encompasses not only the nutrients we consume, but also the environmental repercussions of our food production. Adhering to a clean eating regimen promotes the establishment of a dependable and socially-aware food chain, effectively addressing various concerns such as genetically modified organisms (GMOs), the proliferation of diverse health issues, and the emergence of antibiotic-resistant bacteria.

Consume Whole Nutritional Items

Consume food in its raw, unprocessed form.

Consume food items that do not possess a label indicating their ingredients.

Consume unaltered food products that have not undergone any form of modification.

Please refer to the article titled "Approaches to Maintain a Healthy Diet according to Counteractive Action's Article 23."

Perused Fixing Marks

In the event that there is a labeling indicating its ingredients, it should only display a sole ingredient, such as quinoa.

Refrain from the inclusion of any additives, including but not limited to sugar, salt, vitamins/minerals.

When acquiring bread, it is essential that the label indicates the presence of 100% Whole Grain.

Opt for organic food options whenever feasible.

Opt for meats derived from pasture-raised animals rather than those fed a grain-based diet.

If one is unable to discern the composition of a culinary item, one should abstain from consuming it.

Create Your Means of Survival

It is the most effective method for understanding its contents.

Wholesome food items necessitate minimal preparation.

Any dish you prepare will offer far greater benefits than opting for take-out meals.

Eat Oftentimes

Consume three small dinners and 1-2 snacks per day.

Include protein, carbohydrates, and essential fats in every meal.

You will maintain an optimal blood sugar level for your health.

You shall not experience hunger.

If you exert effort and strive to ascertain the means by which to consume nutritious foods, you will be rewarded with positive outcomes for your physical well-being.

Quinoa And Red Beets In The Mediterranean Style

Ingredients:

- 2 tbsp. of lemon juice - divided
- 1 cup of parsley - chopped
- 1 cup of walnuts - toasted, chopped
- ¼ tsp. of sea salt
- ¼ tsp. of pepper
- Balsamic vinegar
- 6 tbsp. of feta cheese - crumbles
- 1 cup of Quinoa - Rinsed
- 2 tbsp. of olive oil
- 3 cups of red beets - peeled, diced

- 1 bunch of green onions - sliced, divided white and green parts

- 2 tbsp. of garlic - minced

- 1 tbsp. of lemon zest - minced

Instructions:

In a spacious skillet, prepare the quinoa in accordance with the guidelines provided on the packaging. Transfer it to a separate receptacle and set it aside.

On the same skillet, heat your oil over medium-high heat. Incorporate the beets and the onion's white sections. Continue cooking them in a sauté pan until the beets have reached a desired tenderness that allows for easy piercing with a fork. The process is estimated to require a duration of 10 minutes. Incorporate the garlic and sauté it for a duration of 60 seconds. Incorporate the quinoa, onion greens, zest, and juice by gently mixing. Incorporate the parsley and the walnuts. Ensure proper seasoning by adding the salt, vinegar, and pepper. Adorn it with a tablespoon. of feta cheese.

Delectable Culinary Creations
Suitable For Every Dining Occasion

Pancakes

2 tablespoons corn starch

3 tablespoons sugar

2 teaspoons vanilla

1 pinch of salt

1.5 cups flour

1 cup milk mixed with 1 tablespoon apple cider vinegar

2 bananas

2 teaspoons baking powder

This particular recipe is highly effective if one possesses an electric griddle, as it enables a significant reduction in cooking duration.

It is advisable to allow the bananas to undergo a process of counter-ripening until the peels exhibit a streaked appearance of brown and black. By no means decomposed, rather allow them to ripen slightly further. Completely pulverize them in a sizable mixing bowl, subsequently incorporating the milk and vanilla. Blend the components together, subsequently setting them aside.

Combine the dry ingredients before incorporating the mixture of banana and milk. Continuously agitate the mixture until all components have blended uniformly and attained a coherent consistency. Once the griddle has been lubricated with oil, proceed to fill a ¼ cup dry measure by spooning the mixture into it. Carefully inclined the measuring instrument above the cooking surface, gently contouring the edges with the utensil, subsequently ensuring a uniform surface for your pancake. Once the bubbling at the sides becomes notably pronounced, proceed to flip the pancake using a pancake turner with a slim edge. Typically, a standard griddle has the capacity to cook 6-8 items simultaneously. This recipe yields approximately twelve exquisite pancakes, which in my humble opinion, will rival any others you have ever tasted. Additionally, feel free to incorporate your preferred assortment of finely diced fruits.

Embarking On A Clean Eating Journey

Prior to delving into the topic of clean eating, it is imperative that we establish a comprehensive definition of this dietary approach. Clean eating primarily involves the consumption of organic or unprocessed food, thereby representing a fundamental approach to nutrition. Individuals who adhere to the principles of clean eating typically refrain from consuming food that undergoes chemical processing and possesses excessive amounts of sugar. In contrast to prevailing perceptions, clean eating transcends being merely a weight-loss regimen; rather, it represents a novel methodology to enhance the quality of one's lifestyle—incrementally, through each nutritiously balanced meal.

The consumption of food has a significant impact on our overall well-being and physiological state. The physical composition of our bodies mirrors the types of nourishment we consume. Incorporating an assortment of nourishing, nutrient-rich, and organically grown foods into our diet will bestow upon our bodies boundless vitality and a radiant complexion. If you desire to achieve weight loss or gain, this dietary approach will assist you in attaining your utmost physical condition.

The Distinction between Clean Eating and Healthy Eating

A subtle differentiation exists between the concept of healthy eating and that of clean eating. Although clean eating can be viewed as a form of healthy eating, it should be noted that healthy eating encompasses more than simply adhering to a clean eating regimen. The practice of healthy eating entails a mindful approach to food consumption, with the aim of mitigating excessive intake of fats and carbohydrates by the body. This approach to dietary consumption does not differentiate between processed and unprocessed food items, which constitutes the fundamental principle of maintaining a clean eating regimen.

In order to maintain a healthy diet, it is necessary to embrace a higher consumption of plant-based foods. Considering the promotion of natural foods through clean eating principles, it would be advisable for you to increase your intake of whole grains, fresh fruits, and vegetables. It is not necessary for one to adopt vegetarianism in order to faithfully adhere to this dietary approach. With the exception of pre-packaged varieties, all types of meat remain permissible for consumption.

Establishing a routine of frequenting meat establishments will ensure the procurement of the highest quality meats. If one lacks expertise in trimming meat or identifying superior cuts, seeking guidance from the butcher is a viable recourse. Additionally, it is imperative to cultivate the practice of thoroughly inspecting nutritional information provided on food packaging in order to adhere to this dietary regimen. We cannot live off of fresh foods alone and you need to be aware of what ingredients are used when you buy processed foods.

When purchasing foods of this kind, it is advisable to opt for those with a lesser number of ingredients. In addition, it is advisable to refrain from consuming foods that have ambiguous ingredient lists or descriptions, as well as those that contain artificial additives and preservatives.

What are the initial steps to begin adopting a clean eating lifestyle?

Modifying an individual's dietary patterns is among the most challenging habits to alter, yet it is not an insurmountable task. The crucial element for achieving a successful transition to a clean eating regimen lies in adopting a gradual and measured approach, refraining from excessive exertion and undue haste. Fortunately, there are methods available to facilitate a more seamless transition.

The initial step you must take is to provide your own elucidation of the concept of clean eating. Which foods do you regard as being hygienic? What foods are off-limits? By inquiring about these fundamental aspects, you will develop a preliminary understanding of the items to be included in your grocery list, strategies for meal planning, and anticipated duration and expenditure for food preparation.

The majority of individuals adhering to this particular dietary approach abstain from consuming white foods (with the exception of fruits and vegetables), such as sugar, flour, rice, bread, and similar items. This is primarily due to the fact that numerous white foods possess elevated levels of carbohydrates and commonly undergo processing and/or refinement procedures. The act of consuming alcohol is also highly discouraged among individuals who adhere to a clean eating lifestyle.

In addition to their elevated sugar and calorie levels, it is customary to steer clear of consumables containing saturated and trans fats. Nevertheless, it is advisable to seek out alternative sources of fats that are more conducive to maintaining a healthier lifestyle, given the body's continued requirement for essential fatty acids (EFAs).

Initially, it may appear as though you are foregoing the consumption of the foods that bring you joy. However, if you have achieved proficiency in the skill of strategizing wholesome meals, you will come to realize that there exists a vast assortment of culinary options that you can revel in. Moreover, you have the option to indulge in a weekly meal from a restaurant as a form of personal indulgence, if desired.

Additionally, after determining your preferred approach to maintaining a nutritious diet, it is imperative to thoroughly remove any unhealthy food items from both your refrigerator and pantry. This presents a wonderful opportunity for you to engage in the practice of reading labels. Please be reminded that if a certain item consists of an extensive compilation of ingredients and constituents that elicit difficulty in pronunciation or unfamiliarity, it is unsuitable for inclusion within your pantry. Select food products that contain a maximum of six ingredients.

Once the refrigerator and pantry have been organized, the subsequent task entails replenishing and arranging the provisions. Prior to embarking on a visit to the grocery store, it is advisable to formulate a comprehensive meal plan. Given the perishable nature of the food items you handle, failure to adequately plan may result in spoilage. Do you harbor an inclination to squander food and financial resources? Upon acquiring all the necessary provisions, it is also advisable to engage in advance food preparation, thus facilitating the process of cooking a wholesome meal throughout the week.

Furthermore, it would be prudent to consider making an investment in a refrigeration unit. Upon adopting the practice of consuming nutritious foods, one shall undoubtedly recognize the advantages of possessing a refrigerator. The possession of this item will prove advantageous in maintaining the freshness of your food, regardless of your location or circumstances.

Finally, it is imperative to maintain a steady pace. I would suggest dedicating a sufficient amount of time to gradually relinquish the habit of consuming unhealthy food. It is unnecessary to relinquish your preference for certain foods in order to maintain a nutritious diet. Please bear in mind that you have the liberty to designate specific days for indulgence, and furthermore, there exist methods by which you can transform customary preferences into healthier alternatives. There is truly no justification for experiencing a sense of deprivation.

In the forthcoming chapter, you will acquire the knowledge and techniques necessary to transform a traditional recipe into a clean eating recipe. Additionally, I have incorporated a food substitution chart that can be utilized to effortlessly transform any recipe into a wholesome alternative.

Baked Egg Benedict

- 1/8 oz. low-fat Monterey Jack cheese, grated

- ½ cup of baby spinach leaves

- 1 pinch each of sea salt & freshly ground black pepper

- ¼ tbsp. fresh tarragon, chopped

- Olive oil cooking spray

- 1 large egg

- 1/8 oz. uncured, extra-lean, cooked ham, diced finely

- ¼ cup 1% milk

- 1 whole-grain English muffin, toasted & split

- ¼ tbsp. organic butter, unsalted

- ¼ tbsp. brown rice flour

Adjust the oven temperature to 375°F and commence preheating. Simmer the water in a saucepan or kettle until it reaches its boiling point. Mist a 4-oz. Coat the ramekin with cooking spray and position it within a baking pan that measures 9x9", filled halfway with boiling water (if desired, hot tap water may be used as a substitute.) Proceed to crack an egg into the ramekin and add the ham. Permit the contents to rest in the pan until they have cooled marginally. Heat butter over medium heat in a saucepan of medium size until melted. Incorporate the flour into the mixture and cook it for approximately 45 seconds, continuously whisking throughout the process. Add milk gradually. Please continue to whisk the mixture until it reaches a thicker consistency or for approximately 2 minutes. Put off the heat. Incorporate the cheese and gently agitate until it is fully liquefied. Incorporate the salt and pepper by gently stirring, then proceed to set it aside. Preheat a sauté pan on a medium-high heat setting. Combine the water with the spinach. Continuously stir and sauté until the spinach has become wilted, typically taking around 1 minute. Drain. Place the spinach atop the muffin. Gently dislodge the egg by gliding a knife along the interior of the ramekin. Transfer the egg-ham mixture onto the bed of spinach. Incorporate the tarragon into the cheese mixture. Agitate and carefully pour onto the egg and ham mixture. Serve warm.

The Adversary Of The Clean Eating Dietary Regimen

Having acquired an understanding of calorie counting in relation to basal metabolic rate (BMR) and activity metabolic rate (AMR), as well as gaining insight into the correct balance of carbohydrates and fats, you likely have discerned the rationale behind the multitude of issues associated with various fad diets.

The majority of dietary regimens are likely to be ineffective as they prioritize immediate results, thereby neglecting the essential long-term aspect of preserving the body's equilibrium.

Initially, we examined the adverse effects of a low-fat diet, as an excessive focus on carbohydrates leads to a temporary surge in energy followed by a subsequent decline due to a sugar crash.

It has come to our attention that hunger arises from a depletion of our serotonin levels, thereby triggering an unconscious drive to seek expeditious means of bolstering both our serotonin and energy reserves. The ultimate objective is to commence the consumption of carbohydrates such as chips, crackers, or candy as a means to satisfy one's snacking desires.

In this chapter, I aim to elaborate further on the detrimental pattern wherein the consumption of carbohydrates leads to a subsequent crash in blood sugar levels, followed by a tendency to snack on additional carbohydrates that ultimately results in another blood sugar crash. I characterize this recurring pattern of consuming carbohydrates followed by energy crashes as a deterrent to adhering to a clean eating dietary regimen.

The crucial aspect in breaking free from this detrimental cycle pertains entirely to the influence of serotonin on our hunger response.

Currently, depression is commonly examined alongside serotonin. Within that particular framework, it is designated as the neurotransmitter associated with positive emotions. An optimum or elevated degree of it is correlated with a sensation of contentment and an elevated state of tranquility.

On the opposite side of the spectrum, diminished serotonin levels are associated with depression, anxiety, or apprehension.

Serotonin is a topic that arises infrequently in discussions centered around the subject of nutritious food choices. Moreover, the majority of individuals are unaware of the extent to which consuming a well-rounded meal influences their snacking habits and satiety level.

Nonetheless, serotonin plays a crucial role in the regulation of appetite as it governs our degree of satiety, dictating the level of contentment our body derives from the quantity of nourishment it has ingested.

Serotonin plays a pivotal role in communicating satiety signals to the brain, effectively signaling the cessation of further food consumption.

Serotonin carries out its physiological functions by means of the ingestion of carbohydrates. Virtually all carbohydrates will possess a certain quantity of tryptophan. Tryptophan, an amino acid, is additionally found within protein.

Consuming carbohydrates leads to a significant increase of tryptophan in the bloodstream. The tryptophan will circulate within your bloodstream until it is fully depleted by your body.

Provided that there is an adequate presence of tryptophan within your system, upon the activation of your body's insulin response, your bodily functions will commence the assimilation of essential nutrients, thereafter transforming them into usable energy.

This sequence of events will result in an excess of tryptophan, subsequently initiating its circulation within the brain. Tryptophan offers the fundamental constituents necessary for the synthesis of serotonin in the body.

Therefore, upon reaching the brain, the tryptophan undergoes conversion into serotonin, culminating in the ultimate outcome.

By this point, I presume you possess a significantly enhanced understanding of the rationale behind categorizing certain cuisine as comfort food, as well as the tendency for certain individuals to express irritability in the face of hunger.

The phenomenon of experiencing elevated mood after consuming a meal rich in tryptophan, and the subsequent decrease in mood associated with a sudden decline in blood sugar levels, can be elucidated by the interaction between carbohydrate-induced sugar crashes and the conversion of tryptophan into serotonin.

The remarkable aspect is that you now possess the knowledge to address the feeling of being irritable due to hunger in a manner that adheres to the principles of clean eating.

In fact, the cycle of tryptophan converting to serotonin is just one of multiple digestive functions that the body employs to communicate satiety to the brain.

Another mechanism that is employed to indicate satiety is through the utilization of Leptin, which serves as an additional hormone.

Leptin is synthesized by the gastric glands. Similar to other neurosoma and endocrine substances, Leptin communicates to the brain the signal of satiety and the need to terminate the act of consumption.

The primary objective of examining these various digestive processes and the subsequent communication between the brain and body, whether it be regarding satiety signals or energy depletion, is to emphasize the critical significance of maintaining a well-balanced dietary regimen.

When addressing our dietary habits, the sole means by which we can govern our biology is through the regulation of our consumption. Assuming we adhere to a well-rounded nutritional regimen encompassing diverse and wholesome foods, it is generally feasible to sustain our desired weight and experience a sense of well-being, owing to the inherent workings of Serotonin, unless we suffer from a hormonal or similar medical ailment.

Nevertheless, it remains a fact that unless you partake in well-rounded meals comprising various food groups, you will persist in experiencing the detrimental consequences associated with fad or unhealthy dietary trends.

What constitutes the primary adversary of a diet plan centered around clean eating? It comprises commercially purchased snacks and quick-service restaurant solutions.

If an individual persists in consuming a diet predominantly comprised of processed food snacks, the outcome will be an inundation of sugar into the bloodstream, consequently leading to the perpetuation of the detrimental cycle of snacking followed by subsequent energy crashes as expounded upon in the earlier section of this chapter.

Indulging in unhealthy or processed snacks necessitates frequent subsequent snacking. You will experience fleeting satiety, but steadily accumulate weight.

The phenomenon of experiencing a drop in energy levels after consuming sugar, followed by consuming unhealthy snacks, highlights the inability of your body to promptly utilize the immediate burst of energy obtained from these sources. The sole foreseeable consequence is the accumulation of surplus energy in the form of adipose tissue.

One can solely regulate their inherent digestive processes by exercising control over the substances one introduces into the system. In essence, that encapsulates the essence of clean eating.

Consume a well-rounded diet and allow the body to maintain a naturally slender physique, providing us with an optimal level of vitality to sustain ourselves throughout the day.

I consistently advocate for the inclusion of complex carbohydrates in a dietary regimen, as opposed to endorsing a diet plan that completely eradicates complex carbs.

In my opinion, excluding complex carbohydrates from one's dietary intake is predisposing oneself to potential difficulties. Incorporating complex carbohydrates into one's diet entails the consumption of food items such as rye bread, sweet potatoes, and various vegetables.

Replace those food categories with alternatives such as vegetable-based snacks or whole grain options, including whole wheat bread and whole grain pasta. Utilize the knowledge acquired from this chapter regarding the adversary of maintaining a wholesome diet, in a calculated manner, in order to effectively curb hunger pangs and resist the temptation of consuming processed or unhealthy foods.

The foremost piece of advice I would like to offer is straightforward in nature. In the event that you experience intense hunger, it is advisable to consume a modest portion of easily digestible carbohydrates in combination with a small portion of complex carbohydrates.

The minimal quantity of simple carbohydrates will sustain your satiety until your body initiates the digestion of the complex carbohydrates. This advice will assist in accelerating the sensation of satiety, without precipitating any detrimental consequences commonly associated with the rapid increase and subsequent drop in blood sugar levels resulting from carbohydrate consumption.

Nevertheless, provided your caloric intake remains relatively stable and aligned with your plan, it is unlikely that you will experience sensations of hunger between meals once your personalized clean eating diet plan is well-adjusted to your AMR. This exemplifies the genuine magnificence of adhering to a healthy dietary regimen.

Processed snakes, junk food, and certain dietary regimens are also adversaries of clean eating as they typically lack the essential nutrients required by the body to sustain an optimal level of physical well-being, while providing only a momentary surge of sugar.

If you have ever come across discussions regarding vacant calories, it originates from this very concept.

It is conceivable that one could sustain oneself and potentially achieve weight loss by exclusively consuming products made from white bread.

Nevertheless, consuming this would result in a significant intake of nearly 100 percent devoid of nutritional value. Even if you were to achieve weight loss through the implementation of a white bread diet regimen (an approach I strongly advise against), it is important to note that attaining physical fitness is not guaranteed.

Due to the lack of protein intake, your body would be unable to develop muscle tissue, thereby rendering you physically unfit. Furthermore, the absence of essential vitamins and minerals would impede the promotion of overall bodily health and cognitive strength. The deficiency of imperative nutrients required to regulate hormone levels may result in an unfavorable mood. Consequently, by depriving your body of its fundamental nutritional requirements, you would be neglecting its utmost necessities.

The notion of empty calories extends beyond the context of a white bread dietary regimen, encompassing various prepared meals, fast food diets, as well as processed foods available in packaged forms such as boxes or cans.

There exists a myriad of issues linked to the consumption of an imbalanced diet.

The most unfavorable scenario is the consumption of a diet consisting solely of empty calories. Insufficient intake of essential nutrients can result in an increased appetite, potentially contributing to weight gain, impaired health, and diminished energy levels.

The rationale underlying the concept of clean eating revolves around placing confidence in one's own body.

Our physical bodies possess an inherent ability to perceive which foods are essential, and upon receiving the necessary nutrients, our bodies will communicate this by prompting us to consume those specific foods.

Prevent consumption of nutrient-deficient foods by adhering to a 21 day regimen focused on consuming whole and nourishing meals.

After the completion of a 21-day regimen focused on clean eating, you will acquire a profound understanding of your body's signals and requirements for maintaining optimal fitness and a lean physique.

The adherence to a diet based on whole, unprocessed foods will furnish you with ample energy and a surge of beneficial hormones, ensuring a well-rounded, flourishing and physically alert existence.

Stew Consisting Of Chickpeas, Sweet Potatoes, And Spinach.

- 1 teaspoon fresh grated ginger

- 1/2 teaspoon turmeric

- 1/2 teaspoon cumin

- 1 tablespoon curry

- Salt and pepper, to taste

- Pinch red pepper flakes, optional

- Cilantro, to taste and for garnish

- 2 (19 ounce) cans chickpeas, rinsed and drained

- 2 (28 ounce) cans whole tomatoes, including juice

- 2 onions, chopped

- 1 sweet potato, peeled and cubed into 1 inch pieces

- 6 cloves of garlic, crushed and minced fine

- 2 cups packed baby spinach

On a stovetop set to medium heat, utilize a spacious skillet to sauté onions in a modest amount of olive oil until they attain a tender consistency, which typically takes approximately 5 minutes. Incorporate the curry, turmeric, cumin, garlic, ginger, salt, and pepper into the mixture; stir and continue to sauté for an additional 1 to 2 minutes.

Simultaneously, heat the diced sweet potato in the microwave, without covering it, for approximately 4 to 5 minutes, taking into consideration the size of the cubes. Agitate intermittently to guarantee uniform cooking.

Incorporate the chickpeas and tomatoes into the mixture and proceed to mix it together. Reduce heat to a gentle simmer and place a lid on the pot for a duration of 10 minutes. (Include the sweet potatoes once they have reached a state of tenderness that can easily be tested with a fork.)

Detach the cover and incorporate a maximum of 1/4 cup of water into the mixture (adjusting to achieve your preferred thickness). Simmer 5 minutes more.

Remove from heat and incorporate spinach until it becomes wilted. Garnish with cilantro.

Crunchy Quinoa Granola

- 1/4 Teaspoon Ground Nutmeg

- 1/4 Cup Unsweetened Applesauce

- 1 Teaspoon Vanilla Extract

- 2 Tablespoons Raw Honey, Melted

- 1 Egg White

- Cooking Spray

- 1/2 Cups Uncooked Quinoa

- 1/2 Cup Rolled Oats

- 1/4 Cup Unsalted Shelled Pumpkin Seeds (Pepitas)

- 1/4 Cup Dried Cherries

- 1/4 Unsweetened Shredded Coconut

- 2 Tablespoons Chia Seeds

- 1/2 Teaspoon Ground Ginger

- 1/2 Teaspoon Ground Cinnamon

Set the oven temperature to 300° F prior to use.

Position a baking sheet with rim dimensions of 9 x 13 inches onto a sheet of parchment paper.

Combine raw quinoa, coconut shreds, chia seeds, pumpkin seeds, cinnamon, rolled oats, dried cherries, and nutmeg in a mixing bowl.

Incorporate honey, applesauce, and vanilla.

Whisk the egg in a bowl until it becomes foamy, then incorporate it into the mixture with quinoa.

Distribute quinoa evenly on a baking sheet.

Apply a fine mist of cooking spray onto the surface of the granola, then proceed to bake it for a duration of 45-50 minutes.

Retrieve from the oven and allow it to cool.

Place within a hermetically sealed container.

Chicken And Mustard Sauce

¾ c. chicken broth

¼ tsp. pepper

3/8 tsp. salt

4 chicken breasts

2 Tbsp. olive oil

12 oz. Brussels sprouts

1 Tbsp. parsley

2 Tbsp. butter

2 Tbsp. Dijon mustard

¼ c. apple cider

Directions:

Please set the oven temperature to 450 degrees.

Whilst that is being heated, proceed to heat a skillet with a small amount of oil. Prior to placing in the pan, it is essential to season the dish with a sprinkle of pepper and salt. Cook for a duration of 3 minutes, rotate and subsequently transfer the pan into the oven.

Set the timer and allow the baking process to proceed for approximately 9 minutes. Remove from the pan while ensuring it remains heated. Proceed to warm the pan, followed by the introduction of ½ cup of the broth and the cider. Begin by heating the mixture until it reaches its boiling point, then adjust the temperature to a lower setting and allow it to simmer for a duration of 4 minutes. After this, proceed to include the parsley, 1 tablespoon of butter, and mustard.

Proceed to heat the remaining butter and oil in a separate skillet, subsequently introducing the Brussels sprouts into the pan. Cook over medium heat for a duration of 2 minutes and subsequently incorporate the remaining broth and salt. Continue cooking for an additional duration of 4 minutes.

Present all of the mixtures simultaneously and relish the experience.

Okinawa Diet Seaweed-Infused Broth

Ingredients

1 teaspoon minced fresh ginger

1 tablespoon miso

3 scallions, chopped for garnish

4 -5 cups water

5 inch pieces of kelp or 5 inches of Kombu

1/3 cup dried shiitake mushrooms or 1/3 cup other dried mushroom

Directions

Heat water to boiling in saucepan.

Add in kelp.

Add in dried mushrooms.

Allow to simmer for 60 minutes

Take out mushrooms, and sea veggies and dice and bring back to pot.

After this, add in ginger and allow to simmer for ¼ hour.

Mix in miso. Use the scallions as garnish.

Dietary Regimens Inspired By The Clean Eating Philosophy

Numerous diet programs have derived their structure from the principles of clean eating, albeit not all of its pertinent methods have been implemented. Below are a few examples of popular diet trends that closely adhere to the principles of clean eating:

The Raw Food Diet

The raw food diet emerged during the initial years of the 1980s as a potential remedy for the cholera epidemic, which was believed to have been partly exacerbated by the cooking techniques employed by individuals. The proponents of this dietary approach maintain that unprocessed elements possess an elevated nutritional profile, a substantial portion of which is assumed to be compromised during the culinary preparation. They also place greater emphasis on organic foods, particularly those that have not undergone industrial processing, as they perceive them to be more valuable. Additionally, they hold the belief that the application of heat, particularly when oils are utilized, gives rise to noxious substances that have adverse effects on an individual's well-being. Preservation is achieved through refrigeration, without the need for cooking or the use of chemicals.

The raw food diet is commonly denoted as raw foodism. As suggested by its nomenclature, the focus lies on the consumption of food articles in their intrinsic state, requiring minimal or absence of preparation or cooking. It promotes the practice of avoiding the consumption of the majority of processed foods, similar to the concept of clean eating. However, it imposes restrictions on the types of food that individuals can consume due to the prohibition on cooking.

The program encompasses the intake of a variety of fruits and vegetables, nuts and seeds, fish, meat, dairy, and fresh eggs. Dairy products that have been subjected to the processes of pasteurization and homogenization are strictly prohibited. The sole types of processed foods permissible for consumption by individuals adhering to a raw food diet encompass yogurt, kefir, kombucha, cheese, and sauerkraut.

The Paleo Diet

The Paleo diet, derived from the eating habits of prehistoric humans, encompasses principles that align with the notion of consuming nutritious foods in their unprocessed form. According to popular belief, this dietary approach is acclaimed for its ability to assist individuals in maintaining a slender, high-energy, and overall robust physical condition. With backing from research conducted across multiple scientific disciplines, the Paleo diet, akin to the concept of clean eating, underscores the deleterious impact of contemporary processed foods on the human body.

The diet primarily focuses on the ingestion of lean proteins, fruits, vegetables, seafood, nuts and seeds, and wholesome fats. It advocates for refraining from consuming dairy, grains, processed food, sugar, legumes, starches, and alcohol. These limitations demonstrate the subtle disparities between the Paleo and clean eating approaches, with the latter emphasizing the inclusion of whole grains in one's daily dietary regimen.

The Comprehensive Nine and Thirty-Day Lifestyle

A program of relatively recent inception, the Whole 9 and Whole 30 lifestyles have emerged as offshoots of the Paleo diet, integrating various techniques that foster psychological well-being into this regimen. The range of permissible foods is more limited, yet the emphasis still lies on enhancing one's well-being, resilience, and overall vigor.

The numbers 9 and 30 are associated with the set of factors that the creators have identified as significant in attaining a harmonious state of mind and body. Illustrations of such are temperance, socialism, slumber, and the management of stress.

Purifying And Balancing The Physical System

What does the term 'Alkaline Cleanse' denote?

An alkaline cleanse can be described as an approach that entails restricting the intake of cooked food and beverages, while focusing exclusively on the consumption of uncooked, fresh soups, smoothies, and juices which are abundant in alkaline content. This method is typically employed for a span of 3 to 10 days, although certain individuals may opt to extend the duration beyond the initial 10-day period. The primary goal of this procedure is to eliminate the accumulation of harmful substances within the body through the administration of readily assimilated, alkaline-based nutrients. This facilitates a comprehensive purging and regeneration of the blood, tissues, and organs across all bodily systems.

To recapitulate, throughout an alkaline cleanse, you provide your body with a comprehensive array of essential nutrients in a manner that facilitates convenient accessibility and absorption, specifically through the utilization of a liquid medium. Simultaneously, you conscientiously refrain from any exposure or interaction with substances that are detrimental to the well-being of the body.

This may appear to be a challenging and demanding procedure, necessitating a restriction of the usual content one usually requires. However, in reality, the opposite is true. In the course of an alkaline cleanse, one eliminates superfluous chemicals and substitutes them with a substantial infusion of nutrients, calories, and liquefied sustenance. This dietary plan does not involve fasting; therefore, you are free to consume a substantial amount of nutritious food at any time. Should you experience hunger, simply avail yourself of additional servings.

Is there any other matter that should be considered?

Another crucial element of a cleanse regimen is consuming a substantial amount of water. More precisely, this implies the provision of high-quality, sanitized, and refined water. Additionally, you have the option to enjoy herbal teas or warm lemon water to add variety to your beverage choices.

What are the substances or factors that one refrains from consuming or engaging in while undertaking an alkaline cleanse?

To put it succinctly, the only things you need to be concerned with are fresh, organic, uncooked alkaline juices, smoothies, and soups. As long as you adhere to these choices, there is no imperative to possess an exhaustive inventory of the numerous substances and ingredients you will be excluding. However, for individuals new to the alkaline cleanse, it may be of interest to familiarize yourself with certain key restrictions that must be consistently avoided in order to achieve optimal results during your Detox.

In the absence of a specific sequence, presented herein is an inventory of sustenance to refrain from during the process of purging and enhancing alkalinity:

Saturated fats

Trans fats

Crisps

Sugar

Chocolate

Fizzy drinks

Bread

Yeasts

Corn

White pasta, rice, and noodles, among others

Simple carbohydrates

Mushrooms

Fruits with elevated sugar content (choose lemons, limes, grapefruit, avocado, tomato)

Alcohol

Tobacco

Dairy

Fresh eggs

Meat

Refined foods

Frozen foods

Fermented foods

Condiments

Caffeine

Microwaved foods

Have you considered the utilization of nutritional supplements?

Supplements hold the same level of significance during a cleanse as they do in your everyday life. They are exclusively intended to augment a well-rounded diet, rather than serving as a substitute. Supplement usage should only be considered in the event that one's regular diet and beverage intake fail to sufficiently provide a particular nutrient. As long as the products utilized are of natural origin and devoid of toxins, they will not compromise the integrity of your cleanse. There exist several recommended supplements for an alkaline cleanse that are advised to guarantee the absence of any potential complications with regard to your dietary intake:

By ingesting a substantial quantity of fluids, you inadvertently forgo a portion of the dietary fiber typically obtained through the consumption of solid sustenance. The inclusion of a natural fiber supplement will prove highly advantageous in aiding the detoxification process of your gastrointestinal tract, thereby facilitating enhanced absorption of vital nutrients from the wholesome, uncontaminated substances you are ingesting. Fiber supplements are highly recommended within the context of an alkaline cleanse, and their utilization can greatly enhance the efficacy of your cleanse.

The utilization of a natural, herbal-based supplement designed for the purpose of parasite cleansing, known as a Parasite Cleanse product, offers a commendable method for eliminating the unexpectedly prevalent quantity of parasitic organisms within your bodily system. Additionally, the herbal nutrients contribute to the facilitation of a comprehensive purification of the digestive system, aiding in the elimination of accumulated deposits of mucus, yeast, and waste substances. Conduct thorough research to identify a suitable parasite cleanser that can aid in facilitating your Detoxification process.

Crucial Fatty Acids: It is imperative to consistently include Omega 3, 6, and 9 fatty acids in your daily diet, despite the notable challenge in doing so. Surprisingly, these essential nutrients are recognized for their elusive nature through dietary sources alone. Research suggests that a substantial 70% of the global population faces chronic inadequacy of these vital substances, with a particular emphasis on Omega 3. This insufficiency can give rise to various minor complications in our everyday existence. While undergoing a cleanse, it is of heightened significance to incorporate these oils into our dietary regimen as they do not hinder the detoxification process, but instead offer us a pristine and effective means of obtaining energy. Seek out natural supplements that encompass all three vital fatty acids to aid in your detoxification process, and contemplate perpetuating their utilization even upon completion of the cleanse.

Green (Wheatgrass) Powder: This dietary supplement can serve as an agent that expedites the detoxification process during an alkaline cleanse. They exhibit a high concentration of essential nutrients that will thoroughly nourish the body and facilitate its healing and regeneration processes. If one desires to maximize the benefits derived from an alkaline cleanse, the process of rejuvenation free from the influence of toxins becomes indispensable, amplifying its efficacy can undeniably prove advantageous.

Possessing an alkaline nature, it is imperative during the detoxification process to ensure an intake of approximately 4 liters of water per day. However, it is of utmost significance that the water consumed for this purpose be not only alkalizing, but also uncontaminated, devoid of the very toxins one strives diligently to eliminate. Incorporating pH drops into the water that you ingest is an effective means of maintaining a pH level of approximately 8-9, thereby guaranteeing that the water possesses an optimal degree of alkalinity for the purpose of facilitating your cleansing regimen. Truly, this tool is imperative for achieving a successful cleanse.

Is it advisable to engage in physical activity during an alkaline cleanse?

Indeed! Participating in physical activity during the cleansing process is highly advantageous. Nevertheless, it is essential to engage in aerobic exercises, prioritizing cardiovascular activities, rather than anaerobic exercises such as weightlifting or resistance training. Engaging in excessive physical exertion is ill-advised, especially if you do not adequately consume the requisite quantities of carbohydrates and proteins required for muscle recovery and development during weight lifting. Engage in low-impact exercises such as brisk walking, gentle jogging, or swimming, avoiding excessive exertion.

Engaging in aerobic exercise facilitates the elimination of toxins from the body by purging them through perspiration, respiration, and lymphatic drainage, whereby lymph, a transparent fluid abundant in white blood cells that purify the body's tissues, flows into the bloodstream via the lymphatic system. In the event of excessive exertion, one may encounter symptoms such as lightheadedness and fatigue, which impede certain bodily processes essential for the facilitation of detoxification. Moreover, engaging in anaerobic exercise can trigger the production of specific acids that align precisely with the chemicals one seeks to steer clear of during an alkaline cleanse.

Please bear in mind that the primary aim is to ensure optimal facilitation of self-healing. Taking this into consideration, adhere to physical activities that facilitate this process, while refraining from engaging in actions that may impede or obstruct it.

The Tenets Of Nutritious Consumption

Clean eating entails directing one's attention towards the consumption of nutritious, natural, and minimally manipulated food options. Although the name may be unfamiliar to you, its principles are based on widely recognized and efficacious methods of healthy living. It is a rudimentary notion, yet one that yields significant advantages. The primary objective of this approach is not centered around quantifying caloric intake or eliminating specific food categories. Instead, the emphasis is placed on relishing in the consumption of fresh foods that provide the optimal nutritional value. Hence, it is regarded as a means to adopt a more salubrious way of life, gradually and steadily. The following are the emphasized principles of clean eating:

Opt for unprocessed, whole foods and minimize the consumption of processed food items.

Opt for unprocessed options rather than processed ones.

Be vigilant in monitoring your intake of sugar, fat, and salt at all times.

Consume a total of four to six meals throughout the course of the day.

Refrain from consuming beverages with high calorie content, such as coffee and soft drinks.

Eliminate refined sugar.

Acquire the necessary skills to prepare your own sustenance.

Incorporate a balance of lean protein and complex carbohydrates into each of your meals.

Avoid alcohol.

The Relationship Between Nutritional Intake and Weight Management

By practicing a clean eating approach, it becomes feasible to effortlessly prioritize six small meals within the span of a day, ensuring that they are spaced out at regular intervals of approximately 2 1/2 to 3 hours. This aids in the regulation of blood sugar levels, typically associated with weight gain, and enhances metabolic function throughout the day.

Adhering to a regimen of healthy eating practices will allow you to steer clear of processed food items, such as snacks, potato chips, cookies, pastries, carbonated beverages, and more. In doing so, you facilitate the effortless maintenance of a balanced body weight.

Consuming freshly harvested vegetables and fruits contributes to optimal bodily equilibrium, providing essential nutrients that promote overall wellness and physical fitness.

Clean eating promotes the consumption of low-fat proteins and complex carbohydrates in every meal you partake in. By engaging in this practice, you establish a composite of nutrients that can be efficiently assimilated by your body.

Maintaining optimal health and physical fitness can be achieved solely by incorporating beneficial fats into your diet. When adhering to the clean eating regimen, one will come to recognize the utmost significance and indispensability of incorporating healthy fats into their diet, such as those derived from sources like avocado and fish.

Consuming water is advised as part of a clean eating regimen, and it is advisable to aim for a daily intake of approximately 4-6 glasses. Water is a crucial element in the process of weight reduction as it accelerates metabolism and sustains vitality, thereby augmenting physical exertion.

Breakfast holds significant importance in one's daily routine, and adhering to the principles of clean eating necessitates prioritizing this meal on a consistent basis. Failure to consume breakfast often leads to an inclination towards unhealthy food cravings throughout the day, or even excessive intake during subsequent meals. This leads to an augmentation in overall body weight and adipose tissue.

Consuming your evening meal at least three hours prior to bedtime facilitates the calorie-burning process within your body, thereby promoting sustained vitality and physical well-being.

In the realm of clean eating, the significance of portion control is consistently underscored, as vigilantly monitoring the quantities of all food groups in your meals will ultimately enable you to maintain an optimal weight.

The types of food to refrain from consuming

Saturated fatty acids and trans fatty acids.

Alcohol.

Artificial sweeteners.

Sugary drinks.

Excessively prepared meals, especially those containing refined flour and sugar.

High-calorie sustenance lacking in nutritional value.

Foods with additives.

Artificial food items, such as processed cheese slices, serve as exemplars.

Food products containing a blend of chemical compounds such as artificial food dyes and sodium nitrite.

CHAPTER TWO

DIETARY RECOMMENDATIONS: FOODS TO OMIT

Dietary recommendations and prohibited food items for maintaining a clean eating regimen

1. Maintain distance from items that were produced in manufacturing facilities.

This encompasses all varieties of unhealthy food and a majority of processed food options. Ice cream, sausages, ketchup, breakfast cereals, confectionery, pizzas, low-fat dairy products, and numerous other items. It is advisable to assess whether the appearance of the food you are about to consume closely resembles its natural state. If that is not the case, then it is likely that you have no desire to consume it. This rule does admit some exceptions, including high-fat dairy, which is regarded as beneficial due to its substantial vitamin K2 content.

2. Prefer the option with less processing.

It can prove to be financially burdensome to consistently consume organic food, and it is not obligatory to do so unless one possesses the financial means to afford it. Conversely, there is frequently a healthier alternative that undergoes lesser processing. For instance, in the event that grass-fed beef is economically prohibitive, one could consider opting for grain-fed beef of a reputable brand that exhibits a natural appearance and is minimally enhanced with additives.

3. Eat plants and animals.

During the Paleolithic era, as hunter-gatherers, our sustenance comprised both fauna and flora. It appears to be a rational conclusion that these food items possess the capacity to maintain our overall well-being, given that our physiological composition has been inherently adapted to their consumption. The concept of optimal foraging theory applies in this situation, wherein if the sustenance you are about to consume can be obtained from nature without requiring a substantial amount of time to acquire a nutritionally sufficient meal, then it is likely acceptable to proceed with consuming it.

4. Refrain from consuming food items that contribute to the development of contemporary ailments.

Sugar is the foremost adversary we face, followed closely by processed omega-6 vegetable oils and wheat. If you are capable of eliminating these three foods entirely from your life, then you are already making significant progress towards adopting a nutritious lifestyle. Eliminating these three food items contributes to approximately 80% of the overall health advantages associated with maintaining a nutritious diet.

By adhering to this comprehensive list of minimally processed food options and implementing the accompanying recommendations on foods to be avoided, it can be assured that your overall health will undergo a significant and noteworthy enhancement. The primary factors contributing to contemporary health issues are an imbalanced diet and insufficient physical activity.

Food items to steer clear of within the Clean Eating regimen

All packaged, canned, and processed food and beverages, particularly those that contain additives, preservatives, and other synthetic compounds.

Sandwiches, hamburgers, pizza, whole wheat pasta, sushi, tomato-based sauces, tofu dishes, wheat noodle dishes, any dish that contains Asian soy sauces, baked potato, omelets, egg-based breakfast dishes, wheat and corn tortillas, burritos, empanadas, lattes, cappuccinos, all coffee beverages, and various desserts, except for fruit salad or plain fruit.

Dairy products and fresh eggs: all, including whey and butter alternatives; all types of butter and mayonnaise, including ghee.

Grains: white rice, wheat, corn, barley, spelt, kamut, rye, triticale, oats (including gluten-free varieties)

Fruits and vegetables: oranges, freshly squeezed orange juice, grapefruit, bananas, strawberries, corn, creamy vegetable dishes, nightshade family (including tomatoes, peppers, eggplants, and potatoes).

Animal protein sources include pork (bacon), beef, veal, sausages, cold cuts, canned meats, frankfurters/hot dogs, shellfish, any raw meats, and fish.

Plant-based protein sources include various soybean products such as soy sauce, soybean oil used in processed foods, tempeh, tofu, soy milk, soy yogurt, and textured vegetable protein. Please take note that both miso and fermented soy sauce are indicated as acceptable.

Nuts and seeds: peanuts and peanut butter

Oils: shortening, processed oils, canola oil, the majority of salad dressings and spreads.

Beverages: alcoholic beverages, non-fresh-pressed fruit juices, caffeinated drinks such as coffee and black tea, carbonated soft drinks including low-calorie options, "natural" sodas, or energy drinks.

Sweeteners: white and brown refined sugars, honey, maple syrup, high-fructose corn syrup (HFCS), agave, evaporated cane juice.

Accompaniments: traditional chocolate (containing dairy and sugar), tomato sauce, relish, chutney, most preserves (sweetened with sugar), barbecue sauce, teriyaki sauce, chewing gum, breath fresheners.

A few precautions to be mindful of" or "Several factors requiring caution

Corn starch is frequently found in baking powder, beverages, and processed food items.

Vinegar, mayonnaise, and certain varieties of mustard can be derived from either wheat or corn.

Baked goods marketed as lacking gluten may nonetheless contain oats, spelt, kamut, or rye.

Numerous canned tunas incorporate texturized vegetable protein (TVP), derived from soy. In order to ensure authenticity and avoid adulteration, it is advisable to seek out low-salt alternatives that predominantly consist of unadulterated tuna without any fillers.

Multi-grain rice cakes encompass more than just rice. Kindly ensure the purchase of unadorned brown rice cakes.

The term "natural flavors" has the potential to indicate the presence of monosodium glutamate (MSG).

Numerous amaranth and millet flake cereals incorporate oats or corn.

Make an effort to refrain from using xanthium gum whenever feasible. Guar gum is a preferable option for incorporating fillers, however individuals with heightened sensitivities towards gum additives may not find it suitable.

To ensure optimal results, it is recommended to refrain from or limit the consumption of food items that promote acidity, such as alcohol, various types of beans, beef, chicken, corn, dairy products, fresh eggs, fish, grains, lamb, nuts, pork, plums, prunes, rice, sodas, shellfish, sugar, sweet potatoes, processed tomatoes, turkey, and unripe fruit. Please note that certain food items marked with an asterisk (*) may be consumed in accordance with the provided guidelines.

Exercise caution with regards to these prevalent sources of heavy metal exposure in food and packaging:

Aluminum - cooking utensils made of aluminum, baking powder, containers made of aluminum, dairy products including milk, drinking water, preserved foods, food additives for color, powdered vanilla, table salt, seasonings, bleached flour, American cheese.

Cadmium can be found in sources such as tap water, water from galvanized pipes, carbonated beverages, refined wheat flour, canned evaporated milk, processed foods, and oysters.

Cautionary elements: consumption of water obtained from plumbing systems containing lead, consumption of vegetables grown in soil contaminated with lead, ingestion of canned fruits and juices, consumption of canned evaporated milk, consumption of milk derived from animals that have been fed on lead-contaminated land, consumption of organ meats, and use of eating utensils.

Mercury: Seeds treated with methyl mercury fungicide, predatory fish, and specific lake fish.

Arsenic contamination can be found in various sources, including the presence of insecticide residues on fruits and vegetables, drinking water, well water, seawater, and even wine.

Factors That Indicate Its Suitability For Your Needs

Given the existing evidence, it is irrefutable that adhering to a clean eating lifestyle is accompanied by numerous advantages for one's health. However, individuals may be curious to ascertain the authenticity and personal efficacy of this approach. Indeed, adherence to the aforementioned principles will yield favorable results, as clean eating emphasizes the consumption of well-balanced meals, prudent portion control, and refrains from excluding any food categories, as previously mentioned. The subsequent are supplementary rationales as to why it would be compatible for you:

• It does not aim to cause food deprivation or starvation, instead, it emphasizes the inclusion of nutritious options in your meals.

• You will gain insight into acquiring the appropriate dietary choices

• Implementation of the required changes is feasible regardless of the budgetary constraints.

• Its aim is to foster empowerment and avoid inducing feelings of gloominess.

• The practice of consuming foods that are free from additives and are minimally processed can lead to increased vitality and enhanced overall well-being.

• Adhering to a clean eating regimen will help alleviate bloating.

• It has the potential to promote fat loss and facilitate the reduction of excess body weight.

• Engaging in a nutritionally conscious dietary regimen provides a secure choice for the well-being of your family.

• As it is contingent upon natural food sources, you will not be confronted with processed foods.

• Clean eating is contingent upon the application of logical reasoning.

• The implementation of clean eating is a straightforward endeavor.

• Embracing a clean eating lifestyle will grant you the opportunity to savor the authentic flavors of unprocessed, natural food.

• You will experience a decrease in appetite.

• It is your responsibility to take ownership of the progress you achieve, and it holds you accountable.

• This is a way of living that will enhance your well-being.

A Comprehensive Guide On Making The Transition To Clean Eating: Step-By-Step Process

Consider a situation wherein an individual has been enduring intense abdominal discomfort, excessive gas, queasiness, unintentional weight reduction, chronic fatigue, and various other symptoms, leading to the recent confirmation of a diagnosis of Celiac disease. It is a long-term autoimmune condition, and the physician recommended adhering to a strict gluten-free diet, commonly referred to as 'clean eating'. Indeed, the concept of "clean eating" is indeed being discussed.

Should the individual aforementioned not possess familiarity with the aforementioned nutritious dietary regimen, it is conceivable that they might experience distress, exhibit heightened emotional reactivity, and even contemplate a catastrophic conclusion to the world as they know it. A positive development for them is that transitioning to Clean Eating should be free from any kind of stress, and the entire process is expected to offer them a considerable amount of enjoyment and satisfaction.

While it is inevitable that obstacles will arise, such as your body's resistance to the dietary modifications and potential discomfort associated with them. You should consider it as an opportunity for personal growth, gaining novel insights, and experiencing life from an alternative vantage point as an active participant. "It is imperative for individuals aspiring to pursue a clean eating lifestyle to adhere to the following guidelines:

Determine the underlying reasons behind your desire to embark on this journey.

Embarking on the journey of adopting a clean eating habit necessitates a significant amount of exertion. Consequently, one must engage in profound contemplation regarding the underlying motivations and driving forces behind this endeavor. It is possible that you are experiencing a medical condition that could be alleviated by adhering to a nutritious diet, or perhaps you are intending to enhance your physical fitness for an upcoming athletic competition. It is possible that you are starting to experience apprehension regarding the consequences of your prior unhealthy actions, and you may be genuinely concerned about the potential long-term impacts on your health. As a result, you may be inclined to seek redemption and commit to living a health-conscious lifestyle moving forward.

The aforementioned scenarios provide ample justification for anyone wishing to adopt a healthier dietary regimen. The most compelling catalyst to initiate metamorphosis must originate internally within the individual and is deeply rooted in optimistic mindset.

Determine the Amount of Time You Are Willing to Allocate

Developing new habits aligned with transformative goals can require a considerable amount of time, potentially extending over several months or longer. Once you have determined your rationale, it is crucial that you ascertain the amount of time you are willing to allocate for the purpose of orchestrating your meals, procuring the necessary ingredients, and preparing your culinary delights. Irrespective of one's perspective, striving for a highly nourishing diet is undoubtedly a paramount objective for the vast majority in the long run.

Quick Tip 5

One may opt to forgo their beloved Saturday night television program in order to dedicate time to preparing nutritious breakfasts that could sustain them throughout the entire week.

Conduct a comprehensive evaluation of your current dietary patterns.

By utilizing a culinary log, one can effectively monitor their dietary intake, allowing for a comprehensive assessment of necessary additions as well as potential reductions in their current eating regimen. Upon obtaining the necessary data for your analysis, it will be incumbent upon you to discern any prevailing patterns within your samples, and subsequently compile two lists encompassing: "

• Foods that may not be conducive to a healthy diet that you may consider reducing consumption of; nevertheless, if you possess an extensive inventory of such foods, you could choose approximately 3-5 prominent examples such as foods high in sugar, carbonated beverages, and unhealthy snacks that you would prefer to address as a priority.

Furthermore, you would need to compile a comprehensive inventory of nutritious foods that are currently lacking in your current routine. Please bear in mind that the primary objective of adopting a clean eating approach is to prioritize the consumption of foods that are abundant in essential nutrients, rather than merely reducing the intake of unhealthy options. Additionally, it is prudent to consider the quantity of vegetables on your shopping list. Should any inadequacies arise, you may consider supplementing it with a few additional varieties of vegetables during your next shopping excursion.

• Exercise pragmatism when choosing your objectives.

Once you have determined the unhealthy foods to eliminate from your routine and the nutritious options to incorporate into your dietary plan, you will need to make some strategic decisions. A highly effective and practical approach would be to establish a series of incremental objectives that can be progressively pursued, which is far more advantageous than attempting to tackle the entirety of the task immediately. In this manner, they are able to swiftly calculate the totals. The important inquiries that necessitate consideration are as follows: which adjustments are anticipated to yield the greatest likelihood of achievement? Among the small clean eating habits, which one do you plan to adopt as your initial choice? Commence the new month by incorporating the accumulated amount and proceed accordingly.

Establishing SMART Goals and Documenting Them

It is imperative that you establish objectives that adhere to the SMART criteria, encompassing specificity, measurability, attainability, realism, and timeliness. For example, consider the scenario where you seek to confront your compulsion towards consuming unhealthy, doubly fried donuts. Perhaps you consume approximately four pieces on a daily basis, thereby necessitating the establishment of crucial parameters for your aforementioned objectives.

Initially, it may be necessary for you to establish your objective through the proposition of a self-regulatory statement, such as: "I intend to refrain from consuming copious amounts of donuts."

The aforementioned statement lacks specificity in its objective and fails to address other essential parameters. For instance, it does not specify the quantity of donuts permitted per day, if any are permissible at all. Therefore, it is necessary to further modify the statement as follows: "

I intend to limit my consumption of donuts to a maximum of two per day over the course of the next week. Subsequently, I will proceed to limit my intake to a single donut in the subsequent week while abstaining from consuming any donuts entirely in the subsequent third week. In the event that I feel compelled to consume donuts, I will opt for nutritious homemade snacks (preferably consisting of fruits and vegetables) that have been conveniently stored in my refrigerator. I will accompany these snacks with a plentiful intake of water to satiate my cravings."

The aforementioned statement has presented a set of quantifiable and precise targets, outlining the precise quantity of donuts you aim to reduce on a weekly basis. It also includes a well-defined timeline for achieving these objectives, along with suggestions for incorporating healthier substitutes or alternatives to ensure that these goals are practical and attainable. To achieve this, it is imperative that you dedicate yourself wholeheartedly and conscientiously apply significant effort.

Consequently, there exists no ambiguity in the aforementioned declaration. It provides a straightforward and effective means for managing one's cravings.

The final step entails documenting your objectives and, if feasible, affixing them to the walls of your bedroom or kitchen as a constant visual reminder of the task at hand.

Examine the Nutritional Information on the Labels

Acquiring the ability to comprehend the information presented on food labels is an essential component of adopting a clean eating regimen as it enables individuals to thoroughly ascertain pertinent details concerning the consumables prior to ingestion. It is crucial to bear in mind that not all packaged products pose a risk to one's health. Therefore, it is imperative to carefully scrutinize the ingredients listed on the labels, as this will empower individuals to make well-informed choices. There are several imperative guidelines pertaining to labels that must be adhered to in order to maintain a clean eating regimen, encompassing:

• Prioritize food products labeled with terms such as "modified," "refined," or "hydrolyzed."

• In addition, it is important to be aware of ingredients that contribute to further processing and words that terminate with "ose," as they indicate the inclusion of sugars. One prevalent instance is the term "fructose."

• Endeavor to identify product labels that include terms such as "gluten-free," "whole grains," and "whole wheat" within the listed ingredients. Nevertheless, it is advisable not to make purchases solely based on the presence of these phrases on the products. It would be prudent to conduct thorough research on the products and visit establishments that are well-known for offering natural and minimally processed foods.

• It is imperative to ascertain that food items containing high calorie content predominantly derive their calories from fiber and proteins.

• Ensure that the sodium, saturated fat, and sugar contents indicated on the labels are minimized to the greatest extent possible.

• The labels should list only a limited number of ingredients, and it is important to carefully consider each one. One should approach this task with the question, "Is this ingredient suitable for my kitchen and for consumption?" If the answer is negative, it must be eliminated and an alternative pursued. Indeed, should the contents listed on your product's label exceed a total of five components, it would be prudent to abstain from its purchase, as these substances are unsuitable for inclusion in your shopping cart, culinary space, and digestive system.

• If there is an ingredient on the label that you don't understand, the chances are that you are dealing with a highly processed food, and then you'll have to think about putting it back on the shelf.

In order to assess the proximity of foods to their natural state, one must consider them through the lens of their relationship with the ocean, the land, and the trees.

If the label resembles a scientific composition, it is advisable to refrain from consuming the product.

In my personal opinion, when it comes to selecting ice cream, my preference is for those that possess a low carbohydrate content, are devoid of chemicals, and comprised solely of four ingredients comprising cream, milk, egg yolks, and sugar.

Quick Tip 6

It is imperative to engage in the practice of perusing product labels to scrutinize the listed ingredients, as the terms "organic" and "natural" can occasionally prove to be deceptive.

Purchase in substantial quantities

In order for your clean eating program to achieve success, it is imperative that you secure agreements with grocery stores that possess well-stocked produce and freezer sections, enabling the procurement of food items in large quantities. Acquiring such a store will enable you to stock your freezer with a wide assortment of fruits, vegetables, beef, poultry, and so forth. You shall receive the necessary provisions and be granted immediate access to pre-prepared meals. One can also engage in the practice of procuring items in bulk through online platforms.

Quick Tip 7

Purchasing food items in large quantities preserves two valuable resources, namely time and money (accompanied by noteworthy discounts). These factors contribute to the cost-effectiveness of adopting a clean eating lifestyle.

Furthermore, you have the opportunity to purchase certain food items through online platforms.

Give prominence to a meal or snack at a particular moment.

As previously mentioned, it is imperative that you approach this matter by tackling one meal at a time, rather than attempting extensive modifications that could potentially overwhelm both you and your family in the future. Commence by selecting a nourishing meal or snack and enhance their nutritional value by incorporating clean alternatives, such as substituting corned beef with grass-fed beef. Before long, you would have fully cleared the meal and removed all the unhealthy options.

Please take into consideration that your family may initially express disapproval towards the modifications, however, demonstrate steadfastness and they will gradually become accustomed to the adjustments you have made. Educate your family members regarding your intention to cleanse the meals, emphasizing that it is not simply a dietary choice, but rather a sustainable approach aimed at enhancing their strength and overall health. However, it is advisable not to eliminate all of their preferred food choices simultaneously.

Go Organic!

Does the expense truly justify the investment? This is a frequently encountered inquiry that individuals often pose when advised to incorporate organic foods into their dietary habits. Nevertheless, when considering the enduring health advantages derived from consuming organic food in relation to its cost, one will discern that it is undeniably an expenditure of great value. What potential benefits can be derived from the consumption of organic foods?

Organic foods are devoid of toxins, signifying the absence of pesticides, herbicides, and any chemical substances throughout the entire process of cultivation, harvesting, handling, and storage. While achieving complete organic status for all food items may not be feasible, it is imperative to incorporate certain organic foods into one's diet, such as Apples, Peaches, Grapes, Celery, Potatoes, Cherry tomatoes, and the like.

• Genetically modified organisms (GMOs) are strictly forbidden throughout the entire process of cultivating, harvesting, and processing organic food.

• As previously mentioned, organic foods are devoid of chemical substances, thereby alleviating consumers from the need to ingest any residues that may be present on conventional foods. For example, a significant quantity of chemicals is annually employed in the United States for the cultivation of non-organic crops. When adhering to an organic diet, one consumes food that is devoid of any synthetic chemical substances.

• Conjugated linoleic acid (CLA) and omega-3 fatty acids, two beneficial fats for cardiovascular health, are typically abundant in organically raised meat and milk. Their consumption can greatly contribute to the promotion of heart well-being.

• Organic food is beneficial for expectant and lactating mothers, as non-organic food items contain chemicals that can be transmitted to the child through breastfeeding and during pregnancy.

• Undoubtedly, organic foods are more beneficial for children as they effectively mitigate their exposure to pesticides, thereby resulting in reduced chemical accumulation within their bodies.

• It is indisputable that the flavor of organically cultivated foods surpasses that of those cultivated using chemical methods.

• It enables the cultivation of robust and high-yielding organic livestock, as the animals receive exceptional nourishment and are raised devoid of antibiotics and growth hormones.

Baked Eggs With Chives

Ingredients:

1 tablespoon fresh chives, chopped

1 tablespoon fresh basil, chopped

1 slice melon

Salt and pepper to taste

2 fresh eggs

1 teaspoon butter

2 tablespoons low-fat milk

1 slice whole-grain bread, toasted

Directions:

Please adjust the oven temperature to 350 degrees Fahrenheit. Grab a 6 oz. Coat a ramekin with a non-stick cooking spray.

Break the fresh eggs and transfer their contents into the ramekin. Incorporate milk, basil, and chives. Season to taste.

Please proceed to carefully position the ramekin within the oven and allow it to undergo cooking for a duration of 15 minutes.

Present alongside melon and toast spread with butter.

Enjoy!

Salad Featuring Broad Bean, Fennel, And Pomegranate

Ingredients:

A handful of watercress

Chopped dill

Chopped mint

Chopped parsley

350 grams of broad beans

200 grams of bulghar wheat

200 grams of pomegranate seeds

2 tablespoons of pumpkin seeds

1 fennel bulb

For the dressing:

1 tablespoons of Dijon mustard

Lemon juice and lemon zest

5 tablespoons of extra virgin olive oil

2 tablespoons of cider vinegar

Directions:

Proceed to heat a sufficient quantity of water within a kettle. Simultaneously, deposit the bulghar wheat into a bowl and incorporate a moderate amount of salt. Proceed to transfer the boiling water onto the bowl containing the bulghar wheat. Enclose it with plastic wrap. Allocate ten minutes.

Arrange all of the dressing's ingredients neatly within a diminutive bottle or jar. Secure the lid firmly and vigorously agitate the container in order to thoroughly mix the contents. Subsequently, return to the bulghar wheat with the intention of assessing its cooked state. If any remaining water persists, evacuate it. Proceed with the relocation of the bulghar wheat into a sizable receptacle, subsequently incorporating the fennel, herbs, broad beans, pumpkin seeds, and pomegranate seeds. Combine all the ingredients and incorporate the salad leaves.

Combine all ingredients, gently coat with the dressing, and present for serving.

www.ingramcontent.com/pod-product-compliance
Lightning Source LLC
Chambersburg PA
CBHW071212020426
42333CB00015B/1383